Table of Contents

Introduction

The moment of truth... You bought a book with recipes and you're trying to persuade yourself that it wasn't in vain. You open it and try to find something catchy on the pages. Finally, you get back to the introduction to see if the author has any important words to tell and convince you that your choice was perfect. And so it was☺

This is a recipe-book with zucchini as a main ingredient. It's small and compact. It has twenty five recipes, that is just enough for you to prepare some special and delicious meals, yet very simple and usually quick (you'll see that, having some practice in the kitchen).

The main ingredient in all the dishes is zucchini. Maybe you think it's a strange choice, but it's a perfect one. Apart from being really tasty, the dishes are very healthy and light (it's a really necessary option for women ☺). So, you have a double benefit. To convince you more, here are some facts about this vegetable that are maybe unknown for you.

The nutritional value that a zucchini offers is impressive. It's really low in calories (with only 17 calories per 100 grams) and high in fiber. It has no cholesterol or unhealthy fats. It's also rich in flavonoid antioxidants which help to slow down aging and prevent diseases with their free radical-zapping properties.

Zucchini is also heart-friendly as it has a wonderful source of potassium (it helps to moderate your blood pressure levels and counters the effects of too much sodium). As a fact, a zucchini has more potassium than a banana.

Zucchini is rich in B-complex vitamins, folate, B6, B1, B2, B3, and choline, also there are minerals like zinc and magnesium, iron, manganese and phosphorus.

This list is almost endless. You see that including zucchini into the dishes is a really good way to stay healthy, to have a strong body, and still it gives you the chance to have enjoyable, tasty meals and desserts (so, no sufferings with limiting some types of meals).

The recipes in our book are divided into three main sections – soups, main course and desserts (my favorite part ☺). They are time-saving, but sometimes you need some extra patience (lasagna is a good example, but the result is worth the efforts). All the ingredients are simple and easy to get at the market (it's a necessary option for me, as simple products help you to understand the real taste of the dish).

All the recipes have the list of ingredients and the instructions step-by-step. If you change or miss something, it can change the result a little bit (it depends on the ingredients that are missed). Don't get nervous in this situation (and don't curse me☺), all the recipes were used loads of times and checked (also, mistakes help us to improve your skills better than anything else).

Now, I'm going to finish this long and maybe boring description for you to get to the practice. The main advice from me – cook with good thoughts and in a good spirit. It is the main spice for all the dishes. Enjoy your time cooking and sharing meals with the people you need, or just being on your own. Let's get started ☺

ZUCCHINI CREAM SOUP

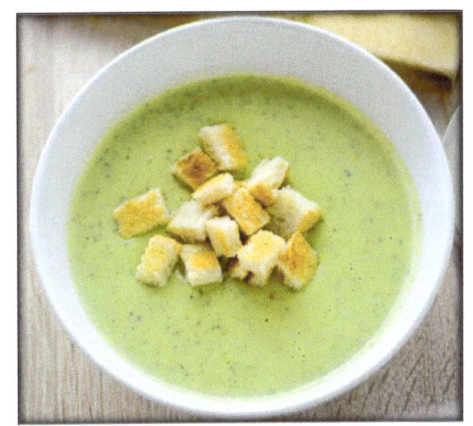

Ingredients:

Unsalted butter - 4 tbsp

Onion – 1 pcs

Garlic - 8-9 large cloves

Zucchini - 4 pcs (medium size)

Chicken or vegetable broth - 4 cups

Fresh lemon juice – 1 tbsp

Salt, pepper, herbs

Instructions:

1. Melt the butter in a pot over medium heat. When it foams, add the sliced garlic and onions and cook on medium-low heat for about 10 minutes (until the onion is soft). The heat should be low enough so that the garlic doesn't get brown.

2. When the onions are soft, add the zucchini and cook until soft.

3. Add the broth and let it simmer for about 45 minutes.

4. Before turning off the heat, add lemon juice.

5. Let it cool slightly, then blend it until creamy (make a puree).

6. Add salt, pepper and herbs (I prefer dill here, but it's up to you).

7. Leave it for some time before serving, so the flavors meld.

8. Serve it with crackers and enjoy-enjoy-enjoy ☺

VEGETABLE SOUP WITH ZUCCHINI

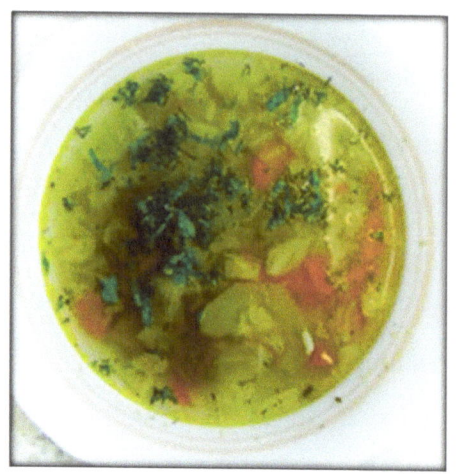

Ingredients:

Zucchini – 1 pcs (middle size, 8-9 oz)

Potato – 2 pcs

Tomato – 2 pcs

Carrot – 1 pcs

Onion – 1-2 pcs

Garlic – 3 cloves

Pepper, salt, dill

Instructions:

1. Boil the water (1-1,5 liters).

2. Peel the potatoes, slice them and add into the water, let it boil for 12-15 min.

3. While potato is being prepared, we'll go in for vegetables.

Slice onion, chop carrot and zucchini (if necessary, peel it and scoop out the seeds).

4. In the frying pan heat the oil. Fry onion first, till it's soft and translucent. Add carrot and fry for 6-9 min more. Then add zucchini and let it stew for 10 min.

5. Peel the tomatoes, chop and add to the vegetables. Stew altogether 5 minutes and turn off the heat. Vegetables are ready.

6. Now, let's get back to the potato. Add the vegetables to it and let everything boil for 5-10 min. We need it to sweat.

7. Almost at the end add salt, pepper and minced garlic.

8. Leave it for some time before serving (10-20 min), so the flavors meld and become stronger.

9. Can be served with sour-cream. Sprinkle the top with the dill.

10. Tasty and light soup is ready. Have a good lunch (or dinner) ☺

SOUP WITH ZUCCHINI AHD MUSHROOMS

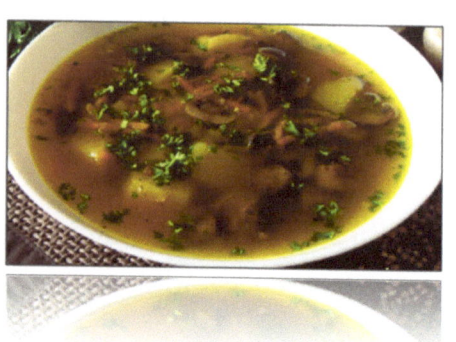

Ingredients:

Zucchini – 2 pcs (middle size)

Mushrooms – 200 g

Potato – 2-3 pcs

Tomato – 2 pcs

Carrot – 1 pcs

Onion – 1 pcs

Unsalted butter – 1 tbsp

Sour-cream – 1 tbsp

Herbs, salt, pepper

Instructions:

1. Cut the mushrooms and boil them during 20-25 minutes.
2. Chop the carrot and onion, sauté them for 10 minutes.
3. Cut the potato and zucchini into dices.
4. After 25 minutes put the carrot and onion to the mushrooms' broth, add potato and zucchini. Keep it simmering during 15-20 minutes.
5. Slice the tomatoes and add them 5 minutes before the end.
6. Add salt, pepper and herbs (if you like them). Often herbs can be used for decoration only, you don't have to eat them.
7. It's better be served hot with sour-cream.
8. Another zucchini soup is ready. Enjoy its taste and your day ☺

ZUCCHINI SOUP WITH APPIES

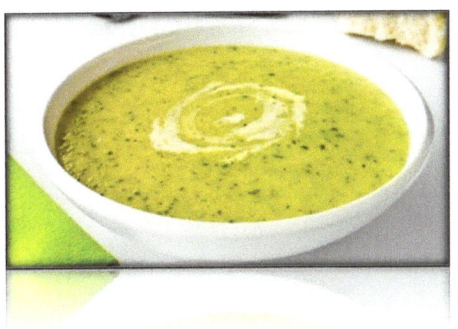

Ingredients:

Vegetable/Chicken broth – 3 cups

Zucchini – 2 cups (chopped)

Apple, celery, carrot – 1 pcs

Crème - ¼ cup

Butter – 1 tbsp

Salt

Instructions:

1. Chop the celery and the carrot, fry them for 10 minutes in the frying-pan in the butter.
2. Peel the zucchinis, cut into pieces, add to the frying vegetables.
3. Boil the broth, add there the vegetables, add salt.
4. Let the soup simmer for 10-12 minutes.
5. Slice the apple, add to the soup, boil everything for 10-15 minutes.
6. Grind the soup in blender to puree and pour back to the saucepan.
7. Add the crème, turn off the heat.
8. Wait 10 minutes before serving.
9. You can decorate this soup with sour-cream on top.
10. Bon appetit! ☺

POTATO WITH ZUCCHINI

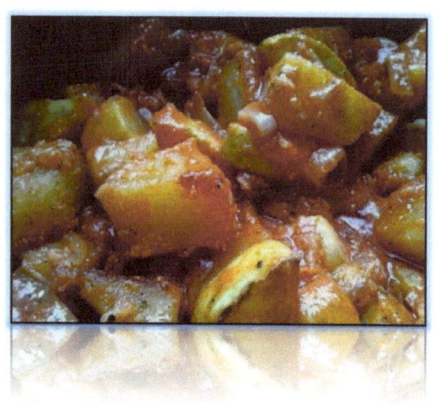

Ingredients:

Potato – 2 pounds

Zucchini – 2 pcs

Onion – 2 pcs

Garlic – 2-3 cloves

Onions – 3 pcs

Tomato paste – ½ cup

Water – ½ cup

Oil

Pepper, salt, herbs

Instructions:

1. Slice the onion and fry a little in the oil till it's translucent and soft.

2. Peel zucchini, scoop the seeds (if necessary); peel the potato and chop everything.

3. In the stew-pan mix onion, potato and zucchini. Add water. Let it simmer for 15 minutes (till it's almost ready).

4. Add tomato paste, minced garlic and herbs.

5. Turn off the heat and let the dish draw for 20 minutes.

6. Serve it with sour-cream, or with fresh tomatoes.

7. This dish is definitely worth trying! Enjoy its taste and lightness! ☺

ZUCCHINI PANCAKES

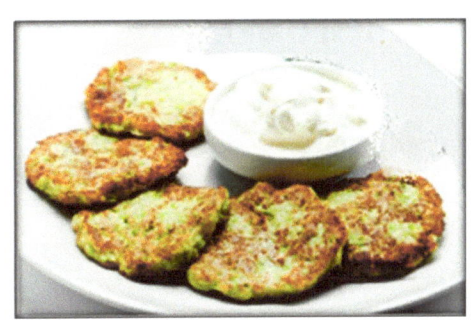

Ingredients:

Zucchini - 3 pcs (grated)

Flour - 1/4 cup

Cheese - 1/4 cup (grated)

Garlic - 2 cloves (minced)

Egg - 1 pcs

Oil, pepper, salt

Instructions:

1. Wash zucchini and trim the ends, grate it and squeeze hard, so there is no juice left.

2. In the bowl sift the flour, add salt and pepper.

3. Beat up the eggs, add garlic and cheese.

4. Combine eggs with flour mix and stir everything.

5. Heat the oil in a large skillet over medium high heat. Scoop tablespoons of batter for each pancake, flatten them with a spatula.

6. Pancakes are cooked until the underside is nicely golden brown, about 2 minutes. Flip and cook on the other side, about 1-2 minutes longer.

7. Pancakes are the best when served at once. It taste will go well with sour-cream.

8. Buen provecho ☺

ZUCCHINI OMELET

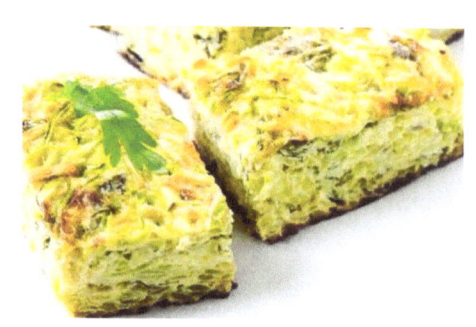

Ingredients:

Cottage cheese – 100 g

Eggs – 2 pcs

Egg white – 2 pcs

Zucchini – 1 pcs

Salt, pepper, parsley

Instructions:

1. Preheat the oven to 350 degrees F (175 degrees C).

2. Peel the zucchini, scoop out the seeds, if they're big, and grate it. Squeeze the flesh, so there is no juice.

3. Beat up eggs till the thick foam, join in cottage cheese, and continue beating.

4. Combine all the ingredients, stir everything, add salt and pepper.

5. Oil the form and pour out the batter into it.

6. Bake it for 20-25 minutes.

7. Serve it hot. You can decorate it with parsley (or dill, tomatoes – it's up to you).

8. Light, easy and quick omelet is ready. Have a good meal ☺

ZUCCHINI LASAGNA

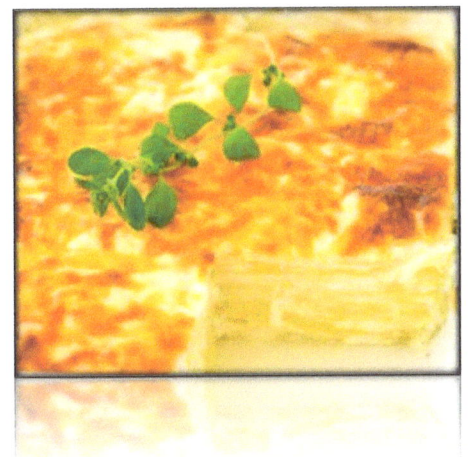

Ingredients:

Tomato Sauce:

Fresh tomatoes - 4 pounds

Garlic - 1 large clove (minced)

Fennel seed – 1tbsp (crushed slightly)

Oregano - 1 tsp (ground)

Basil - 1/4 cup (finely chopped)

Sugar - 1 tsp

Oil - 2 tbsp

Cheese Filling:

Cottage cheese – 1 pound

Cheese - 1 cup (grated)

Egg - 1 pcs

Salt and Pepper to taste

Vegetables:

Zucchini - 2-3 pcs (medium-sized)

Salt - 2 tsp.

Olive oil - 3 tbsp

Mushrooms - 1 pound (sliced)

Spinach - 1 bunch (about 4 cups, chopped)

Onion - 1 large (minced)

Flour - 2 tbsp

Fresh basil leaves (optional)

Mozzarella - 4 cups or 1 pound (shredded)

Instructions:

1. Wash and trim the ends of the zucchinis. Slice them lengthwise to between 1/8 to 1/4 inch thick.

2. Put the zucchinis into a colander and sprinkle the 2 tsp of salt on them. Leave them for about 30 minutes. After 30 minutes, squeeze gently with your fingers each piece, so there is no water. Put the slices on a clean towel and pat the zucchini very dry. Oil an extra-large baking sheet (or 2 smaller ones) and place the zucchini slices in a single layer. Roast in a 375F oven for about 10 minutes. Allow to cool.

3. Deseed the tomatoes (if you wish remove the skins). Bring the tomatoes to a boil and add the minced garlic, chopped basil, crushed fennel seeds, ground oregano, olive oil, sugar, and salt to taste.

4. Simmer everything until thick and reduced (may take up to an hour).

5. In a large skillet heat 2 tbsp of oil and sauté the onions for 3 to 4 minutes. Add the mushrooms and continue cooking. When the mushrooms are soft, add the chopped spinach. When it is cooked, remove from heat and drain any. Add 2 Tbsp flour to the mixture and mix well.

6. Now, let's combine all the layers.

- Oil a 9 x 13 inch lasagna dish and spread about 1/3 of your sauce on the bottom.

- Add a layer of roasted zucchini covering the tomato sauce.

- Add the cheese and cottage cheese mixture and spread evenly.

- Add one more layer of zucchini slices.

- Add a second round of tomato sauce and spread evenly, followed by the vegetable mixture and half of the shredded mozzarella cheese.

- Add the last layer of zucchini slices followed by the third and last round of tomato sauce.

- Place the basil leaves on top of the sauce and sprinkle the rest of the shredded mozzarella on top.

7. Place a baking tray on the rack beneath the lasagna pan, so the juice falling from the lasagna won't get burnt. Bake for about 40 minutes at 350F until the cheese is melted.

8. After it's baked, let it cool.

9. Serve as a separate dish with some fresh tomatoes (it's optional).

10. Enjoy this incredible taste and flavor ☺

BAKED CHICKEN BREAST WITH ZUCCHINI AND TOMATO

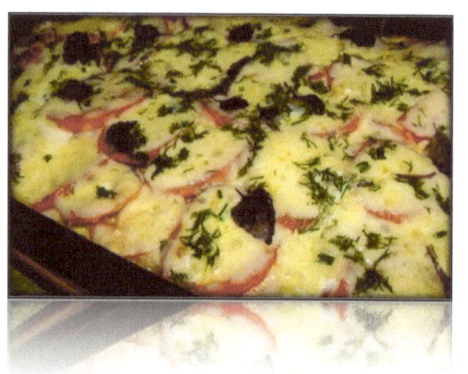

Ingredients:

Chicken breast fillets - 4 pcs (better skinless)

Zucchini - 1 medium

Tomatoes – 2 pcs

Cheese - ¼ cup (grated)

Salt, pepper, paprika

Garlic – 1 clove (minced)

Dill - ¼ tsp

Basil - ¼ tsp

Oil - 1 tbsp

Instructions:

1. Preheat the oven to 170°C/340°F.

2. Wash all the vegetables and cut them into thick slices - 1 inch. Join the zucchini slices with salt and pepper and put them aside.

3. Wash the chicken breast fillets, slice them and rub with salt, pepper, paprika and garlic.

4. Heat 1 tbsp of oil in a skillet on medium heat. Add the chicken breasts and cook both sides for 5-7 minutes, until the meat gets white.

5. Grease an ovenproof dish and place the seasoned chicken breasts into dish. Put a slice of tomato on the chicken, then a slice of zucchini, repeat it.

6. Sprinkle the top with the grated cheese and ¼ teaspoon of dill and basil.

7. Place the dish in the oven for 20-25 minutes, until the cheese on top of the baked chicken is golden brown.

8. It's better be served at once with mashed potato or salad (can be rice – it's up to you).

9. Nutritious, healthy and tasty meal is ready. Bon appétit!

ZUCCHINI IN BATTER

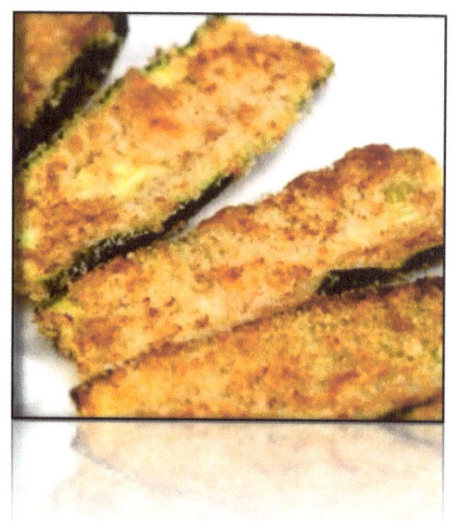

Ingredients:

Zucchini - 3 pcs (middle size)

Eggs - 1-2 pcs (from zucchini size)

Unsweetened yogurt - 100 ml

Flour – 5-6 tbsp

Salt, pepper, garlic powder (optional)

Oil for frying

Instructions:

1. Wash the zucchinis, slice them lengthwise thinly.

2. Season the slices with salt and pepper, optionally you can add a pinch of garlic powder (for better taste).

3. Now batter. Beat the eggs with salt, add the yogurt and flour (4-5 tbsp). The batter shouldn't be very thick, otherwise it will be hard to fry the zucchinis.

4. In one bowl you have sliced zucchini, in another – batted, and the remains of flour – 1-2 tbsp.

5. Take a skillet, heat the oil.

6. Dip a slice into the flour, then into the batter. Fry on both sides for 1-2 minutes – till it gets golden brown.

7. Zucchinis are ready.

8. Serve them hot with sour-cream or garlic sauce.

9. Bon appétit!

BAKED ZUCCHINI PUDDING

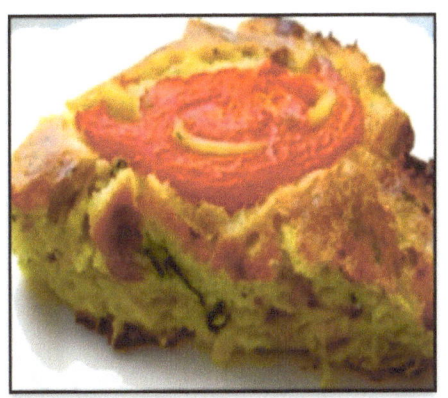

Ingredients:

Zucchini - 3 pcs

Cheese – 100-150 g

Tomato – 2-3 pcs

Sour-cream – 150 ml

Flour - 4 tbsp

Semolina - 6 tbsp

Species, pepper, salt

Instructions:

1. Preheat the oven to 170-180°C/340-360°F.

2. Wash all the vegetables. Grate the zucchinis.

3. Season them with salt, so they will give away extra juice. After 5 minutes squeeze hard.

4. In another bowl, combine sour cream with spices, flour and salt (1/2 tsp). Add this batter to the squeezed zucchinis. Stir everything really well.

5. Add semolina and stir again.

6. Grate the cheese, stir in the batter (3/4 of it). It should be really thick by this time.

7. Oil the baking dish (or cover the bottom with the foil) and pour onto it the zucchini batter. Flatten the top.

8. Slice the tomatoes and put on top, sprinkle everything with the remaining cheese.

9. Bake it for 40-50 minutes.

10. Serve as a separate dish, warm or cooled.

11. Enjoy the combination of flavors in this delicious pudding ☺

SAUTE WITH ZUCCHINI AND VEGETABLES

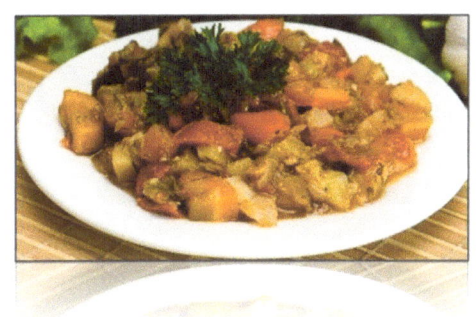

Ingredients:

Zucchini – 2 pcs

Carrot – 1 pcs

Tomato – 1-2 pcs

Onion – 1-2 pcs

Peppers – 2 pcs

Herbs, black pepper, salt

Garlic – 2 cloves

Lemon juice – 1 tbsp

Instructions:

1. Wash all the vegetables. Prepare a stew-pan.

2. Grate the tomatoes. Cut the vegetables into dices.

3. As carrot is the hardest from all, it goes first to the stew-pan with preheated oil. Give it 5-6 min to become soft (cover the pan with the lid).

4. Add onions and minced garlic. 1-2 min will be enough at this stage. Add tomato puree.

5. When all the vegetables are well-stirred, add sliced zucchini, salt, pepper, and stew for 15 minutes everything.

6. At the end, add the herbs and sprinkle it with lemon juice.

7. The dish is almost ready. Don't serve it at once, leave it for 15-20 minutes. All the vegetables will soak the flavor and juice of each other. The taste will become several times better.

8. Serve it as any type of the meal, but don't forget to share it with your family or friends. They'll appreciate it.

9. Enjoy every piece of it ☺

STUFFED ZUCCHINI (VEGETARIAN VARIANT)

Ingredients:

Zucchini – 2 pcs

Peppers – 1-2 pcs (middle size)

Mushrooms – 7 oz

Rice – 2-3 tbsp

Onion – 2 pcs (Middle size. In case you like a taste of fried onion – take more)

Cheese

A pinch of black pepper, salt

Instructions:

1. Preheat oven to 350 degrees F (175 degrees C).
2. Wash zucchini, trim the ends and scoop the flesh out of them.
3. Now the filling. Chop the onions, fry them a little.
4. While frying the onions, prepare the mushrooms. Chop them finely and add to the onions.
5. Cut the peppers and the zucchini flesh. Add to the frying pan.
6. Stew everything till the vegetables are almost ready. Add some salt and a pinch of black pepper.
7. Prepare the rice and add to the vegetables. Our filling is ready.
8. Take the halves of zucchini, stuff them with the filling.
9. Place the zucchini halves into a baking dish, and cover tightly with foil.

10. Bake in the preheated oven for 35-40 minutes, remove from oven, and remove the foil.

11. You can cover the top with grated cheese, it gives a special flavor to the dish and the taste will be better.

12. Another variation of stuffed zucchini is ready. It can be served as any type of meal. Enjoy ☺

STUFFED ZUCCHINI

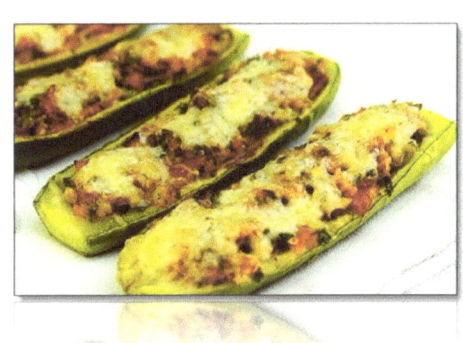

Ingredients:

Ground beef (any other meat) - 1 pound

Zucchini - 2 pcs (ends trimmed)

Bread crumbs – ½ cup

Garlic - 2 cloves (minced)

Black olives

Cheese – ½ cup grated (I use Parmesan)

Instructions:

1. Preheat oven to 350 degrees F (175 degrees C).

2. Cook the meat in a skillet over medium heat until it is browned. Break the meat up into crumbles as it cooks, about 10 minutes.

3. Drain off excess fat, and put the meat into a mixing bowl.

4. Slice the zucchini in half the long way. With a spoon scoop out the flesh, leaving a 1/2-inch thick shell all around the zucchini.

5. Chop the zucchini flesh and add to mixing bowl.

6. Stir in the bread crumbs, garlic, spaghetti sauce, black olives, and Parmesan cheese. Mix everything well.

7. Stuff the halves of the zucchini with the meat mixture. Be attentive, don't press too hard.

8. Place the zucchini halves into a baking dish, and cover tightly with foil.

9. Bake in the preheated oven for 45 minutes, remove from oven, and remove the foil.

10. The stuffed zucchini are ready. Serve them hot or warm. Before serving cover the top with some more cheese, it'll make them look as pizza.

11. Bon appétit ☺

ZUCCHINI WITH APPLES PUDDING

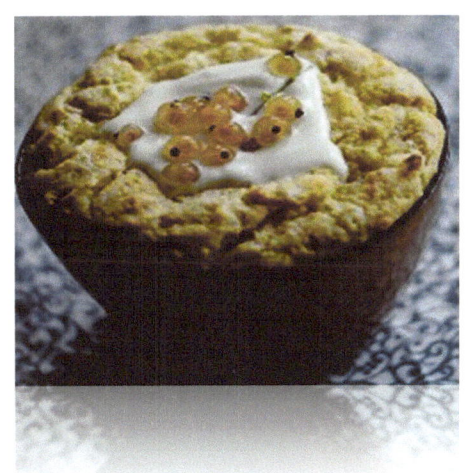

Ingredients:

Zucchini – 11 oz

Green apples – 7 oz

Milk – 100 ml

Butter – 3 tbsp

Eggs – 2 pcs

Sugar – 2 tbsp

Semolina – 4 tbsp

Instructions:

1. Preheat the oven to 350 degrees F (175 degrees C).

2. Peel the zucchini, scoop out the seeds, if they're big, and chop.

3. In a saucepan mix milk with butter, let the butter melt. Add the chopped zucchini, stew until it's almost ready.

4. Peel and chop the apples, add to the zucchini, Add sugar and stew for 5 more minutes.

5. Add semolina and stir well (otherwise it'll have lumps). Cover the saucepan with the lid, stew for 5 more min. Take it away from the oven and let it cool down.

6. Now eggs. Separate yolks from whites. Add yolks to the semolina and mix well. Beat up the whites and then add to the semolina mixture too.

7. Butter the forms, and put there the paste.

8. Bake in the oven for 15-20 min.

9. Light, healthy and tasty summer dessert is ready. Serve it with the crème, add don't forget to decorate it with some berries on top.

10. Yummi-yummi, enjoy ☺

ZUCCHINI MUFFINS WITH CHEESE

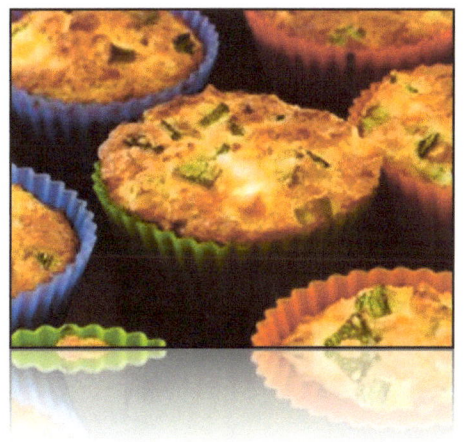

Ingredients:

Flour – 225 g (1 ½ cups)

Baking powder – 3 tsp

Carrot -1 cup (coarsely grated)

Zucchini – 1 cup (coarsely grated)

Cheese – 80 g (1 cup, shredded)

Eggs – 2 pcs

Oil – 80 ml (1/3 cup)

Milk – 125 ml (1/2 cup)

Salt, pepper

Instructions:

1. Preheat the oven to 350-360 F (175-180°C). Line twelve 80ml (1/3-cup) capacity muffin pans with paper cases.

2. Sift the flour and baking powder into a large bowl.

3. Grate zucchini, carrot and cheese. Combine the vegetables and half the cheese. Add salt and pepper, and mix until well combined.

4. Whisk lightly the eggs, milk and oil in a bowl. Add the egg mixture to the flour mixture. Mix until just combined. Finally, add there vegetables with cheese. Stir again.

5. Divide the mixture evenly among the prepared pans and sprinkle with the remaining cheese.

6. Bake in the oven for 25 minutes or until golden. I the cheese on the top got golden brown too quick cover the pan with the foil.

7. Muffins are ready. Enjoy and have a good meal ☺

ZUCCHINI BREAD WITH BANANAS

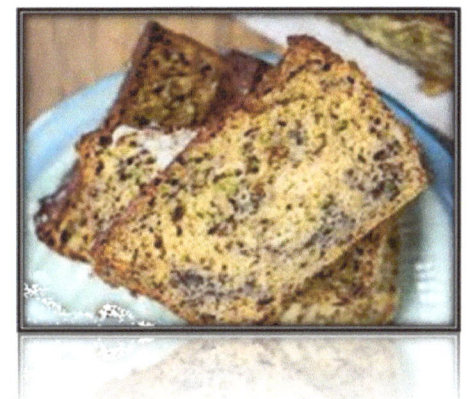

Ingredients:

Oil - 3/4 cup

Eggs – 3 pcs

Sugar – 1 cup

Zucchini – 1 cup (grated)

Bananas – 2 pcs (mashed)

Vanilla extract – ½ teaspoon

Flour – 3 ½ cups

Cinnamon – 1 tbsp (ground)

Baking powder – 2 tsp

Salt – 1 tsp

Raisins, walnuts – ½ cup (each, but optional)

Instructions:

1. Preheat the oven to 325 degrees F (165 degrees C). Oil and flour two 8x4 inch bread loaf pans.

2. In a large bowl, beat eggs until light yellow and frothy. Add oil, sugar, grated zucchini, bananas, and vanilla. Blend everything together until well combined.

3. Stir in the flour, cinnamon, baking powder, baking soda, and salt. Mix in the raisins and nuts.

4. Divide the batter between the two loaf pans, flatter the tops.

5. Bake in the oven about 50 minutes. Check the readiness with a toothpick (insert in the center of the pan, if it comes out clean – the pan is ready).

6. Allow the pan to cool in the loaf pans on a wire rack before removing and serving.

7. This flavor is amazing, try it with coffee or tea, with a scoop of ice-cream or jam.

8. Enjoy ☺

HOMEMADE ICE-CREAM WITH ZUCCHINI JAM

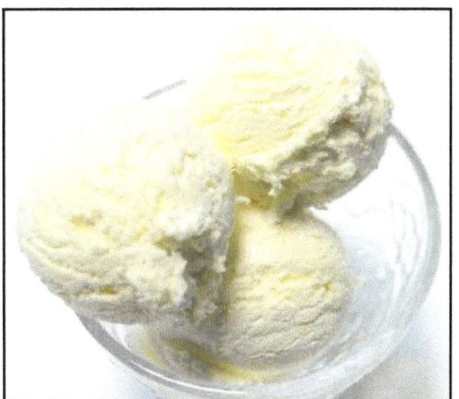

Ingredients:

Sugar – 2 cups

Milk – 1 liter

Unsalted butter – 100 g

Starch – 1 tbsp

Egg yolk – 5 pcs

Instructions:

1. Warm up the milk, dip in the butter. Let it boil.

2. In another bowl, combine sugar, starch and egg yolks. Mix until it has homogeneous and smooth consistency.

3. To this mix add some milk, having it as thick as a sour cream.

4. When the milk starts to boil, pour in the yolk mass, stirring everything all the time.

5. Have it boil and take off from the heat. Put the saucepan into the cold water and stir the mass till it gets cool.

6. Take the special forms (or just plastic glasses) and pour there our ice-cream mass. You can also insert a special stick into the middle.

7. Put everything into the freezer.

8. During a hot sunny day what can be better than homemade ice-cream with jam? ☺

9. Oh, jam is on the next page.

ZUCCHINI JAM

Ingredients:

Zucchini – 2 pounds

Sugar – 200 g (7 oz)

Lemon

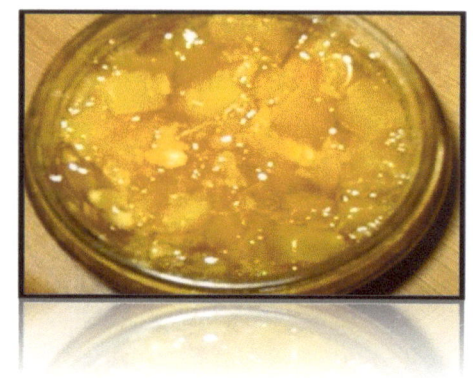

Instructions:

1. Wash and peel the zucchinis. Dessed them. Chop into dices.

2. A lemon zest should be grated separately. Cut into pieces lemon flesh.

3. Add sugar to grated zucchini and in 10 minutes time it will become juicy.

4. Put the zucchinis with sugar on a medium heat, simmer for 45 minutes.

5. Add lemon with zest and keep it on the heat for 15 minutes.

6. Give it some time to rest and simmer everything again until thick and reduced (may take up to an hour).

7. A jam is ready. It's really unusual but tasty. Instead of the lemon, you can use oranges. Zucchinis are good at soaking the flavours, make your own experiments.

8. Serve it with toasts and have a perfect breakfast or snack.

9. Or, take a scoop of the homemade ice-cream (description is above) and several spoons of jam and enjoy your day ☺

ZUCCHINI CAKE

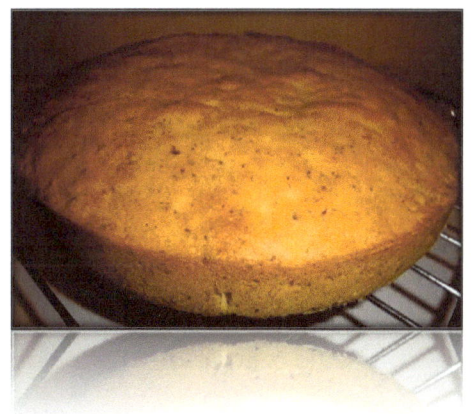

Ingredients:

Zucchini – 1 pound

Starch - 60 g (2-3 oz)

Semolina - 60 g

Unsalted butter - 60 g

Almonds - 100 g

Flour - 50 g

Baking powder - 0.5 tsp

Sugar - 130 g

Powdered sugar - 3 tbsp

Eggs - 3 pcs

Salt

Instructions:

1. Preheat the oven to 170-180°C/340-360°F.

2. Wash, peel and deseed the zucchinis. Cut them into long thin stripes and squeeze hard, so there's no juice.

3. Grind almonds in a blender along with a 1 tbsp of sugar to flour state.

4. In a large bowl, join eggs, salt and the remaining sugar, beat up until a thick foam.

5. Sift the flour with baking powder and starch. Add the flour little by little into a bowl with beaten eggs. Don't stop beating.

6. Melt the butter and pour slowly into a mixture of flour and eggs. Stir well.

7. Add semolina, almond flour, and mix until well combined.

8. Dry zucchini with paper towel, to make sure it has no juice and add into the batter, stir everything carefully.

9. Butter and flour the baking dish. Put the batter onto the form and place into the oven. Bake for 50 minutes.

10. Check the readiness with a toothpick (insert in the center of the pan, if it comes out clean – the pan is ready).

11. Allow the cake to cool on a wire rack before removing and serving.

12. Another variant of zucchini cake is ready. Enjoy it's taste and flavor☺

ZUCCHINI PIE (SWEET)

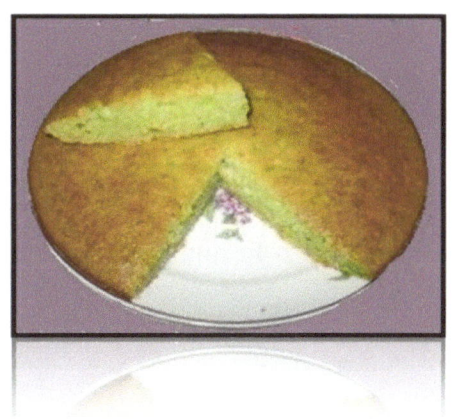

Ingredients:

Grated zucchini - 2 cups

Eggs - 2 pcs

 Sugar -1 and 1/2 cups

Salt - a pinch

Flour - 2 cups

Olive oil - 2 tbsp

Soda - 2 tsp (1.5)

Honey - 2 tbsp (optional)

Vanilla sugar - 1-2 bags (optional)

Instructions:

1. Preheat the oven to 360-390 F.

2. Wash zucchini and, if necessary (in case it's shrunken), remove the peel and the seeds. Grate it and gently squeeze with your hands, measure 2 cups of flesh.

3. Take a bowl, beat the eggs with a pinch of salt, using a fork.

4. Take a bowl with zucchini flesh, add sugar and honey (vanilla sugar), stir everything, wait until melted sugar (about 10 minutes).

5. Join zucchini flesh with eggs and stir everything. Mix soda with vinegar, add to our mixture. Add the flour and knead the dough.

6. Stir everything carefully, so there was no lumps. Add 2 tablespoons of oil.

7. Let the dough "rest" for 10 minutes.

8. Oil the baking dish and cover its bottom with parchment, so that our pie doesn't get burnt.

9. Bake a pie for 30 to 40 minutes.

10. Choose its readiness with a toothpick (dip it into the pie in several places, if it remains clean without pieces of dough, the pie is ready).

11. Cool 10 to 15 minutes before slicing.

12. Serve with vanilla ice-cream, or any type of jam (better to choose a refrigerated one).

13. Perfect delicious pie, a scoop of ice-cream...What can be better during a hot summer day? (And a small amount of calories makes it even more pleasant) ☺

ZUCCHINI PIE (SALTY)

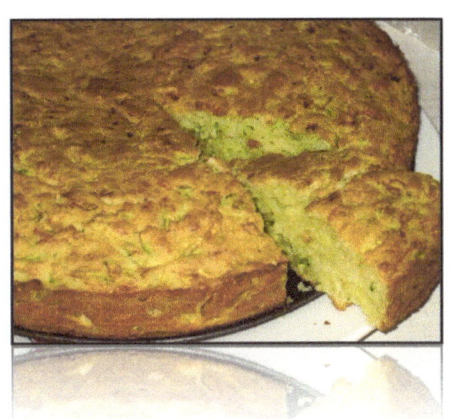

Ingredients:

Zucchini - 2 pcs (middle size)

Tomato – 1 pcs

Flour – 1.5 cups

Eggs - 3 pcs

Salt

Herbs

Cheese - 200 g

Instructions:

1. Preheat the oven to 360-390 F.

2. Wash zucchini and, remove the peel and the seeds. Grate it on the big-holes side of a grater and gently squeeze with your hands, so there is almost no juice.

3. Grate the cheese.

4. Wash the herbs (Parsley and dill are classic variant, but you can add the ones that you like more. Proportion is up to you). Cut them into small.

5. Wash the tomato. Peel it and slice.

6. N.B. If you can't peel the tomato, dip it into a boiling water for as second or two. The skin will be removed quickly after that.

7. In a large bowl, mix grated and squeezed zucchini, 3 eggs, cut herbs. Add the salt. Stir everything together.

8. Now the flour. Add it little by little stirring everything. (It's not necessary to sift the flour before adding to the dough.)

9. Take a detachable baking pan. Oil its bottom and sides, cover it with a parchment. (Make sure, that it covers the sides high enough, so it's easy to take the pie out, when it's ready).

10. Put the dough into the pan. Even the top of it. Put the slices on top. Cover everything with a grated cheese.

11. Put the pie into the oven and bake it for 30 minutes.

12. Leave it for 10-15 minutes in the oven, after its being turned off..

13. It's better to be served warm with a sauce.

14. Easy, light, tasty dinner is ready! Enjoy ☺

ZUCCHINI CHOCOLATE CAKE

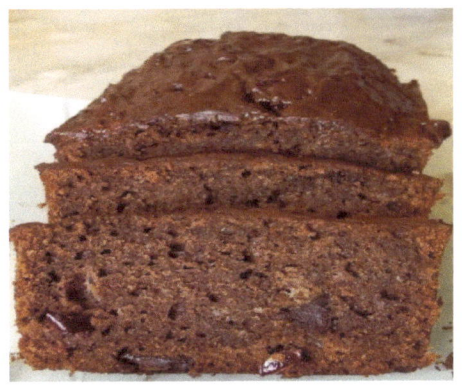

Ingredients:

Zucchini – 2 cups (grated)

Flour – 9 oz

Cocoa powder – 3 tbsp

Eggs – 3 pcs

Sugar – 7 oz

Oil – 200 ml

Baking powder - 1 tsp

Vanilla, sugar powder

Dark chocolate – 100 g

Raisings – ½ cup

Instructions:

1. Preheat the oven to 360-390 F.

2. Wash zucchini and, if necessary (in case it's shrunken), remove the peel and the seeds. Grate it and gently squeeze with your hands, measure 2 cups of flesh.

3. Take a bowl, beat up the eggs, sugar and vanilla. Then, add oil and beat again.

4. Take one more bowl, mix flour, cocoa powder and baking powder. Stir everything well.

5. Chop a bar of chocolate into small pieces.

6. Join zucchini flesh with eggs, flour and raisings. Knead the dough.

7. Stir everything carefully, so there are no lumps.

8. Let the dough "rest" for 10 minutes.

9. Oil the baking dish and cover its bottom with parchment, so that our pie doesn't get burnt.

10. Bake a pie for 30- 40 minutes.

11. Check its readiness with a toothpick (dip it into the pie in several places, if it remains clean without pieces of dough, the pie is ready).

12. Let it cool for 10-20 minutes.

13. Isn't it a strange and delightful combination – tasty and light chocolate cake? Enjoy ☺

ZUCCHINI VANILLA MUFFINS

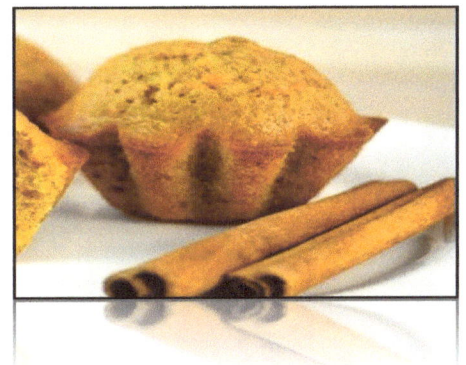

Ingredients:

Grated fresh zucchini - 3 cups

Unsalted butter – 2/3 cup

Sugar - 1 cup

Eggs – 2 pcs

Vanilla - 2 tsp

Baking powder - 2 tsp

Flour - 3 cups

Cinnamon - 2 teaspoons

Nutmeg - 1/2 tsp

Walnuts - 1 cup (optional)

Raisins - 1 cup (optional)

A pinch of salt

Instructions:

1. Preheat the oven to 350°F (175°C).

2. In a large bowl mix the sugar, eggs, and vanilla.

3. Stir in the grated zucchini and then the melted butter.

4. In a separate bowl, mix together the flour, baking soda, nutmeg, cinnamon, and salt. Stir these dry ingredients into the zucchini mixture. Stir in walnuts, raisins or cranberries if using.

5. Take a muffin pan and butter each cup.

6. Distribute the muffin dough equally among the cups, filling the cups up completely.

7. Bake on the middle rack until muffins are golden brown about 20 to 25 minutes.

8. Test with a long toothpick to make sure the center of the muffins are done.

9. Let the muffins cool down and remove from the pan.

10. Muffins can be served with a scoop of ice-cream, with jam, with chocolate or just eaten separately.

11. Don't forget to make a cup of hot chocolate and add a good mood – muffins will taste then even better☺

Conclusion

Ok, we got with you to the end of the book. Some of the recipes were left for better times, some were used and had a great result. I hope you really enjoyed this book and found a lot of useful ideas.

We have only twenty five recipes here, but the real variety is endless. You can change the spices or the fillings and the dish has another taste. Don't be afraid of making your own experiments, I'm sure you'll succeed (even if you need sometimes more the one attempt).

Keep using these recipes, don't forget to give such a treat to your family, relatives and friends as often as you can. Home-made food isn't only healthy and tasty (these are incontestable facts), it creates a special atmosphere at home and in our relationships. The better you have while cooking, the tastier is the food, the better atmosphere and mood you have as a result.

Enjoy your day, see you next time ☺!

science, research, known and unknown facts and internet. The Author and the publisher do not hold any responsibility for errors, omissions or contrary interpretation of the subject matter herein. This book is presented solely for motivational and informational purposes only.

www.ingramcontent.com/pod-product-compliance
Lightning Source LLC
Chambersburg PA
CBHW050836290526
45792CB00001B/413